Top 5 Vitamins and Minerals That Permanently Cure Acid Reflux

Dr Matilda Benjamin

Acid Reflux

Acid Reflux

Acknowledgement

My sincerest appreciation goes out to everyone who has helped me produce "Top 5 Vitamins and Minerals That Permanently Cure Acid Reflux."

I owe a great debt of gratitude to my patients, whose acid reflux problems prompted me to learn more about alternative treatments. The substance of this book would not be what it is without your confidence and willingness to share your experiences.

In addition, I'd want to express my gratitude to the doctors, nurses, and scientists whose ground-breaking research has contributed to our current knowledge of acid reflux and its treatment. Your hard work and devotion to bettering patient outcomes has been invaluable to the writing of this book.

I appreciate everyone's help, advice, and belief in me during this process. Thanks to your knowledge and insight, this book is as accurate and up-to-date as it can be.

Additionally, I'd like to thank my loved ones for always supporting me and believing in me. Thanks to your

encouragement, I've been able to follow my dream of working in holistic medicine and teaching others.
In closing, I want to thank everyone who has bought this book from the bottom of my heart. My honest wish is that you will find some measure of solace from acid reflux here, and that your digestive health will improve as a result. Your determination to improve your health is admirable.

Everyone, I appreciate you being here with me on this amazing adventure. I hope you find this book to be a helpful resource as you work toward intestinal health.

With deep gratitude.

About DOCTOR Matilda BENJAMIN

My name is Doctor Matilda from Los Angeles, USA.
Via my years of experience in my Medical field I've found out that some percentage of people in America and other places around the world is really suffering from Reflux Acid Issues, so I have gone through various viral experiments and experiences which has led me to finally found out the Vitamins that can permanently cure Reflux acid and gives the better life which many people has ever wanted. In this book you will learn all the secrets and vitamins I discovered will permanently cure Reflux acid and the Health tip to help you out in your life journey. I'm so happy that I could be so useful in my years of medical discovery experiences to help out people to get a better life and do well to keep a close eye on my latest medical books to help you much and have a better life.

Acid Reflux

7

Table of contents

NUMBER ONE

NUMBER TWO

NUMBER THREE

NUMBER FOUR

NUMBER FIVE

SIMPLE LIFESTYLE AND HEALTH
HELP TIPS

Top 5 vitamins that permanently cure acid reflux

Acid reflux may be a genuine discomfort, creating a sore throat and an unpleasant sour taste in your mouth; therefore, it is my aim to assist you in controlling acid reflux using natural ingredients like vitamins, minerals, and plants so that you can find long-term relief from this painful condition. Acid reflux can be a real pain; thus, it is my mission to assist you in controlling acid reflux.

It should come as no surprise that up to twenty percent of American adults suffer from acid reflux on an almost weekly basis. If untreated, acid reflux may lead to even more significant health issues.

What Is an Example of Acid Reflux?

Acid reflux, also known as GERD or GASTROESOPHAGEAL reflux disease, is a condition in which stomach acid moves back up into the esophagus, causing uncomfortable symptoms such as heartburn, chest pain, and difficulty swallowing. However, if you take the appropriate steps to manage your acid reflux, you will be able to eat all of your favorite foods without experiencing any discomfort.

The LESS SPHINCTER is a muscular valve that sits at the bottom of your food pipe and just above your stomach. When you eat, the valve opens up and lets food into your stomach, and then it is supposed to close shut to keep stomach acid from going up your esophagus and throat. However, you may be wondering what really causes acid reflux, and the answer is that your stomach produces a lot of acid in order to break down and digest the food that you eat.

On the other hand, this valve may become floppy for certain people, and when they are not swallowing, it doesn't close correctly. When you lie down, stomach acid and digestive enzymes can rise and regurgitate into your food pipe and throat, causing a burning sensation behind your breastbone. Additionally, acid in foods with a sour taste can reflux into your mouth, causing irritation to your throat and making it difficult to swallow. In addition, acid reflux may lower the quality of your sleep and make it difficult for you to function throughout the day. All of this can produce a sore throat and a buildup of mucus, both of which can result in frequent throat clearing and coughing when you first wake up. According to the findings of many studies, acid reflux may often be traced back to an excess of stomach acid. Your stomach's pH should be between 1 and 3, and it is designed to be acidic. However, when the pH level rises to 4 or above, which is more alkaline, the tiny Less valve at the base of your food pipe becomes loose, allowing acid to start flowing back up. The fact that acid reflux can cause major long-term health issues means that it is not only painful; if acid reflux or gerd is not treated, it can result in Ulcer Scars Tissue and damage to your food pipe I am aware that many of you out there take antacid medications in order to treat acid reflux, but the truth of the matter is that this isn't always the best course of action. Although it may provide some relief in the short term, in the long run it may raise the pH of your stomach and neutralize the essential stomach acid, which will make the condition even worse.

WHAT ELSE ARE YOUR OPTIONS THEN?

In this book, we are going to discuss a number of adjustments in lifestyle as well as natural treatments that you may employ to not only put an end to acid reflux for good, but also to bring the pH levels in your stomach back to normal. However, it is important to bear in mind that everyone's situation is different. Before we begin the countdown, it is important to note that consulting your physician before doing anything new is always the best course of action. I would like to take this opportunity to remind you to keep an eye out for any new medical publications that I publish so that you may benefit greatly from the information and expertise that I have to offer.

FRUITS AND OTHER NATURAL REMEDIES

NUMBER ONE

GINGER

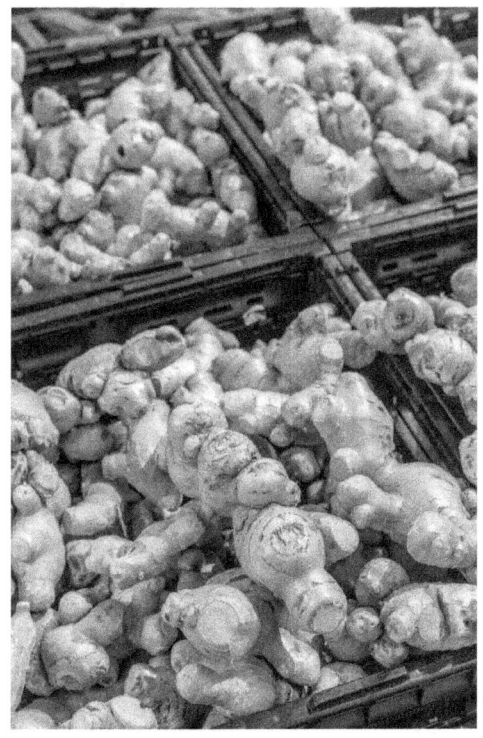

Originating in the countries of Southeast Asia Ginger is a fiery root that is linked to turmeric. The stem of the plant is where the plant's pungent oils are concentrated, making it perfect for use in Ginger Spice. This is why you may hear people refer to ginger as "Ginger Spice." Instead of ginger, it was referred to as ginger root. Acid reflux can prevent us from getting a good night's sleep and is extremely uncomfortable, but don't worry because a piece of fresh ginger root can ease your pain right away. You see, the phenolic chemicals in ginger root can relax the tissues in your esophagus and stomach, reducing the irritation produced by excess acid. If you have acid reflux, try chewing on a piece of fresh ginger root. If ginger extract is taken before meals, it may be possible to experience a reduction in the symptoms of acid reflux that is as high as 40 percent. According to the findings of a research that was recently published in the journal Gastric Disorders and Sciences

Ginger has been shown to have anti-inflammatory properties, as well as the ability to calm tense stomach muscles, stimulate the production of mucus to buffer stomach acid, and reduce inflammation. In addition, ginger has been shown to inhibit the growth of helicobacter pylori bacteria, which has been linked to an increase in the severity of GERD symptoms. Ginger has been used for centuries as a traditional remedy for a variety of health conditions, including digestive disorders.

It is common knowledge that ginger can aid digestion because it stimulates saliva production, which in turn assists the stomach in the process of breaking down food. Furthermore, research indicates that ginger can hasten the process by which the stomach empties into the intestines, which relieves pressure on the lower esophageal sphincter and prevents the reflux of stomach contents into the esophagus. Ginger has been used for several ailments, including indigestion, heartburn, motion sickness, and upset stomachs, for many years. You'll also discover that it has anti-inflammatory and antioxidant properties, both of which will be beneficial to your gastrointestinal tract. After eating, you may take capsules that contain dried ginger powder, but if you want a more natural solution, try peeling fresh ginger and chewing on the root pieces instead. It is beneficial to slice it up and add it to a variety of recipes, including stir-fries, smoothies, and cocktails. We are nearly ready to unveil our top selection of the best vitamins to reduce acid reflux.

NUMBER TWO

APPLE CIDER VINEGAR

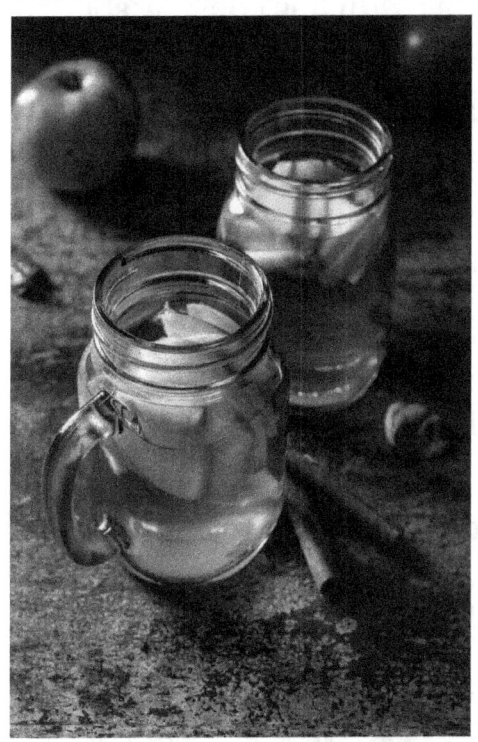

Let's Talk About Apple Cider Vinegar, it all begins with apple juice and yeast which undergo fermentation to create vinegar containing acetic acid and beneficial microorganisms, although this vinegar lacks vitamins minerals or sugar organic versions may contain plant protein strands and antioxidant enzymes but don't be fooled despite its acidity it still has considerable health benefits don't be fooled despite its acidity it still has considerable health benefits Let's Talk About Apple Cider Vinegar, it all In clinical trials, acetic acid was shown to be effective in preventing the growth of harmful germs, reducing inflammation, promoting weight reduction, and maintaining blood sugar levels. A Swedish study found that acetic acid decreases blood sugar levels after meals and slows stomach emptying. Another study found that acetic acid suppresses the action of enzymes involved in the metabolization of glucose. Not only is acetic acid a kind of short-chain fatty acid that gives your colon cells energy and aids in food digestion and nutritional absorption, but it is also a short-chain fatty acid that gives your colon cells energy and aids in food digestion and nutritional absorption. Even though it isn't packed with a lot of nutrients, apple cider vinegar is a powerful source of probiotics that can regulate the intestines and treat indigestion, heartburn, and digestive difficulties. Simply combine one tablespoon of organic raw unfiltered apple cider vinegar with a tall glass of water and sip it via a straw before each meal. By adjusting the pH levels in your stomach, you can improve digestion and ward off GERD and acid reflux. However, for those with an extreme inflammation, If you take two or three apple cider vinegar capsules 30 minutes before each meal, you will discover that this treatment for acid reflux is both straightforward and effective.

Number THREE

ZINC L-CARNOSINE

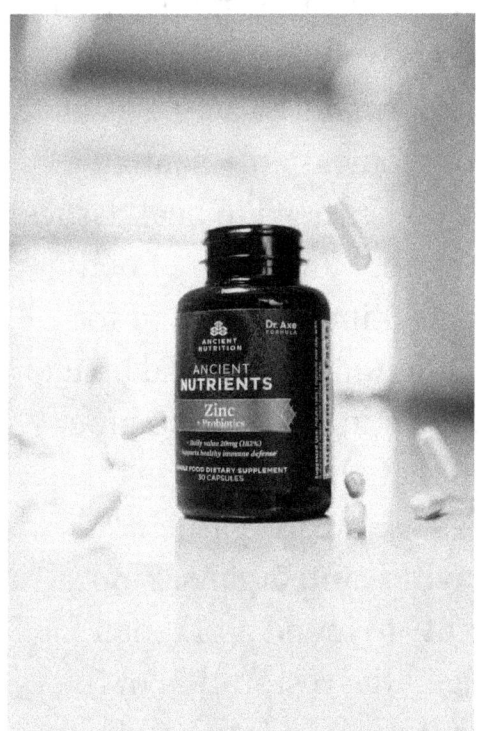

Zinc L-carnosine is a one-of-a-kind combination of zinc and an amino acid named CARNOSINE that has been used as a therapy for acid reflux in Japan since the early 1990s. Studies have shown that zinc L-carnosine may give relief from the uncomfortable symptoms of GERD, such as heartburn and indigestion, by lowering inflammation and preventing stomach acids from hurting the gastrointestinal system. Zinc L-carnosine does this by acting as an anti-inflammatory. Zinc is an essential mineral that our bodies need to heal tissues, particularly the epithelium lining of body cavities and organs. Zinc is also good for treating ulcers, inflammation, and damage to the stomach, intestines, and food pipe. Zinc is a mineral that our bodies use to repair tissues, especially the epithelium lining of body cavities and organs. Zinc aids in the body's ability to mend and repair itself by assisting in the restoration of the mucus barrier that protects the digestive tract. In addition, zinc helps prevent the growth of harmful stomach microbes such as H pylori. The majority of people add 75 milligrams of zinc L-carnosine to their diets each day. However, zinc can also be obtained through the consumption of foods such as shellfish, grass-fed red meat, and pumpkin seeds. Speaking of pumpkin seeds, they are an excellent addition to your diet because just one ounce of them provides approximately 14 percent of your daily required intake for zinc and 37 percent of your

NUMBER FOUR

BETAINE HCL WITH PEPSIN ACID

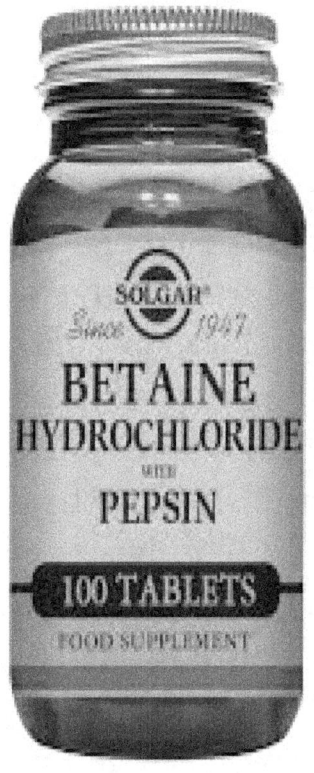

In recent years, researchers have found that

taking pepsin with betaine HCL can reduce the symptoms of acid reflux. Betaine HCL with pepsin is a dietary supplement that has been around since the 1960s. It's thought that the ancient Egyptians used it for therapeutic purposes as well, though they probably didn't know why it works so well to alleviate symptoms of indigestion and heartburn. The symptoms of acid reflux may also be brought on by food that has not been digested coming back up into the esophagus. When proteins and several other dietary components are broken down more rapidly, you may thus reduce the likelihood that this will occur. People who have low stomach acid levels or other gastrointestinal issues may have a difficult time digesting and absorbing protein-rich foods. Because of this, the combination of betaine HCL and pepsin might be helpful as a first stage in the process. Before you can say goodbye to acid reflux for good with this cure, it is essential to seek your doctor's clearance before attempting any new supplements. Try taking two to four 1300 mg betaine HCL Tablets before each meal. Your stomach acid will be replenished, and your digestive system will work properly again. Before you can say goodbye to acid reflux for good with this therapy, however, it is important to receive your doctor's consent.

NUMBER FIVE

PROBIOTIC LIVE BACTERIA AND YEASTS

Live bacteria and yeasts that are known as probiotics are like superheroes for our digestive systems. They play an important part in maintaining an appropriate mix of gut Flora, which in turn supports good health on a systemic level. Yogurt is an excellent source of probiotics. sauerkraut made with kefir Although they may not directly aid digestion, kimchi, miso soup, pickles, and kombucha are all excellent sources of the beneficial bacteria known as probiotics. The gut-brain axis, or the gut's function as a second brain, is responsible for this, and we can thank probiotics for their contribution to brain health by creating neurotransmitters like acetylcholine.

Additionally, probiotics prevent acid from backing up into your stomach, which is one of the other advantages of taking them. Beneficial bacteria in your digestive system stimulate nerves that control the Lesser Esophagus Reflux Disease (GERD), acid reflux, indigestion, and ulcers. syndrome of irritable bowel and gastritis Consuming meals rich in probiotics may help reduce the risk of developing bacterial overgrowth in the small intestine as well as other autoimmune illnesses. medicines related to antibiotics Fermented foods, such as kimchi, sauerkraut, kefir, and pickles, should be consumed regularly to help fix this issue. Artificial sweeteners and fast food meals are also factors that contribute to the reduction of good bacteria in the human stomach. To rapidly build up your microbiota, you may also take a probiotic liquid tablet and drink it with water. This method is just as effective as the high quantities of probiotics that are found in the aforementioned meals.

SIMPLE LIFESTYLE AND HEALTH HELP TIPS

Now that you are aware of the vitamins and natural supplements that have the potential to assist you in permanently putting an end to acid reflux, let's investigate some easy lifestyle alterations that have the potential to assist you in permanently reducing acid reflux to an even greater extent.

1. First and foremost, make some adjustments to your diet by reducing the amount of sugar and vegetable oils you take in. Cut down on your intake of processed foods, which tend to be heavy in things like sugar and salt, and harmful oils. cereals, bread, and biscuits Some of the worst offenders are things like pasta, pastries, and oils like maize, soy, and canola. It is advised that you limit or remove foods like these from your diet while your body is in the

process of healing. Instead of frying or sautéing, consider baking or steaming your food instead. Also, be sure to check food labels so you don't purchase products that have been processed with refined grains and vegetable oils. You can increase the amount of fiber and minerals in your diet by switching from refined grains to whole grains like quinoa, oats, barley, and common wheat. Extra virgin olive oil and avocado oil are both excellent sources of monounsaturated fats, and you should incorporate them both into your diet regularly. Nuts are a good source of polyunsaturated fatty acids. It's also a good idea to include things like pastured eggs, wild salmon and grass-fed butter. Include grilled meats and vegetables that have been steamed in your diet for a natural source of increased energy that your body will reward you for. Modifications to one's way of life

2. Make sure you maintain a healthy weight.

When a person is overweight, their stomach encounters more pressure, which may cause the lower esophageal sphincter (LES) to contract inappropriately, which then leads to GERD since the LES is unable to prevent stomach acid from running back up into the esophagus.

Therefore, to keep one's weight in a healthy range, it is vital to eat healthily and engage in regular physical exercise. On the other hand, processed and fatty foods, as well as alcoholic beverages and caffeine, should be taken in moderation to maintain a healthy diet. Fruits, vegetables, whole grains, and lean meats are all essential components of a healthy diet. In addition to following a nutritious diet, engaging in regular physical activity may help one lose weight and reduce the symptoms of acid reflux. Regular exercise will help strengthen your muscles, particularly those in the lower esophagus, which can minimize the likelihood that you will have acid reflux.

However, you should steer clear of workouts that might potentially trigger acid reflux, such as those that force you to stoop or lay flat on your back, or those that involve continuous jogging or jumping. Consuming a healthy diet and participating in physical activity may help lessen the severity of acid reflux symptoms and lower the risk of developing secondary issues as a consequence of making lifestyle adjustments for GERD.

3. Take care of yourself by practicing self-care. Changing your diet isn't the only thing that can help you keep acid reflux under control. It's recommended, for instance, to avoid eating too close to bedtime. Instead, it's better to eat at least a few hours before going to sleep. Sleeping with your head elevated can also prevent acid from climbing back up your throat.

4. The fourth point is that you may learn to

control your stress through practices like meditation, physical exercise, and quality time spent with loved ones. Outside, extreme stress can cause acid reflux by shutting down the part of the nervous system that regulates calmness and digestion. And that wraps up our top five vitamins that permanently cure acid reflux. We've covered a lot of ground on how to stop acid reflux and GERD and the role of vitamins and natural supplements in achieving this. Remember that it's important to talk to your doctor about what's right for you because everyone's situation is different but incorporating sage, ginger, and turmeric into your diet Therefore, if you put these suggestions into practice, you will be able to regain command of your digestive health and lead a happier, healthier life. Don't forget to keep up with my most recent book releases.

I applaud you for moving forward with putting everything you've learned from this book into practice.